Occupational Medicine

Ashoka Jahnavi Prasad

Contents

Characteristics of Work in Advanced Industrial

Societies Differences in Occupational Cultures
Blue-Collar Workers

White-Collar

Workers Bibliography

OCCUPATIONAL DIFFICULTIES IN ADULTHOOD

Characteristics of Work in Advanced Industrial Societies

The occupational system of advanced industrial societies has certain structural features that appreciably distinguish the work experiences of most persons from those of persons in other types of society. These structural features present the worker with particular types of opportunities. At the same time they confront him with particular types of problems or constraints that affect the quality of his everyday work experiences and relations and the way in which his work fits in with the rest of his personal life and social experience. This chapter is concerned with the social structural sources of strain deriving from occupations.

Work is physically segregated from the home or local residential area. It takes place in a designated workplace to which the worker has to travel because of the concentration there of machines and materials juxtaposed with each other in a planned set of arrangements; an appreciable part of his lifetime (for which no remuneration is received) may be consumed in the journey to work. There is typically little privacy in the work situation; the worker performs before a small "public" and is usually under continuous or intermittent surveillance designed to insure that he meets standards set by his superiors in the quantity and quality of his output. The work is subject to constraints of place, time, and standards set by others. The expression of strong emotion is discouraged. Work is a social activity in which the worker typically interacts with peers, superiors, and subordinates. These exert different types of pressure on him, sometimes conflicting with each other, and he has to manage these in a way that makes his behavior acceptable to all parties. He will be subject to particular pressures to subscribe to the norms of his immediate colleagues in regard to output and to an ideology that attaches special value to their contribution to their employing organization and to society. He must cope with the stresses of dependence and interpersonal conflict, while maintaining enough of his idiosyncratic approach to life to retain his sense of personal identity.

Most work takes place in large bureaucratic organizations. This means that it is done in the name of objectives not necessarily identical with the personal aims of employees; rationalistic means are used to achieve goals; persons are treated as resources available for pursuit of those goals; and subgoals are differentiated into specialized tasks to be performed by specified departments. Tasks are assigned from the point of view of overall efficiency, not from that of the preferences of employees; creativity and innovation are the prerogatives of seniors; rewards tend to be of an extrinsic type (money, space, comfort), rather than being intrinsic to the performance of the task itself, and are related to observed contribution to the overall "organizational" task. Bureaucratic systems of organization facilitate the performance of large scale tasks in mass societies, yield economic and social benefits from specialization and coordination, allocate work to employees systematically on the basis of qualifications, experience, and competence, and help to insure that favoritism and discrimination are minimized. They provide opportunities to many for self-fulfillment in an orderly and progressive career: for colleague- ship, training, advice, and mutual aid. But the ethic of rationalism places the individual at the disposal of his employers, whose requirements may well shift during his work life at points not coincidental with his own needs as these develop.

It is widely assumed or suggested that bureaucracy suppresses individuality. This view has been challenged by recent studies of 3,100 men representative of employees throughout the United States working in similar jobs. Taking organizational size and the number of formal levels of supervision as the main indices of bureaucracy, the results show that those in the more bureaucratic organizations were more likely to be open- minded and receptive to change and tended to value self-direction rather than conformity. They spent their leisure in more intellectually demanding activities. These findings applied to both the public and private spheres of employment and to blue-collar as well as white- collar workers. The researcher attributes the results to three of the occupational effects of bureaucracy: the greater job security of persons working in such organizations, their incomes compared to men of similar educational levels, and the more complex jobs they do. At the same time he notes that bureaucracies provide especially close supervision of staff and that, having hired educated men and given them complex jobs to perform, they may fail to give them as much self-direction as their educational attainments and the needs of the work allow.

When blue-collar workers are considered on their own, smaller subunits are characterized by higher job satisfaction, lower absence rates, lower turnover rates, and fewer labor disputes. The explanation for this is probably that as organizations increase in size and tasks become more specialized, it is more difficult to maintain high cohesiveness or a level of communication felt as satisfactory. These findings do not necessarily imply that largeness of the overall organization in itself determines level of satisfaction, since one can assume, at least in some technologies, that the size of work groups can vary independently of this.

Workers do not choose randomly with respect to the type of firm they join. Those who have a very strong economic orientation have been shown to work for very large companies, and those who emphasize noneconomic factors select the smaller ones. This type of differential selection leads to similar turnover rates in the two types of firms. A separate study of auto workers reports that the men deliberately gave priority to high economic returns at the understood cost of otherwise unrewarding and undemanding work. The majority said they would not be bothered by job changes that would move them away from their current colleagues. Nor did they look to their supervisors for social and psychological support in their work roles.

Large, complex organizations appear to have certain typical forms of psychological stress associated with their functioning. Although most persons, asked whether they would continue to work if this were not financially necessary for them, say they would continue to do so, those in large organizations are especially prone to say they would prefer to do so in a different job or to express significant reservations about what they are doing. Two major stress-producing conditions appear to be the role conflict and role ambiguity, and these appear largely as an outcome of employees' being required to cross organizational boundaries, to produce innovative solutions to nonroutine problems, and to take responsibility for the work of others. No doubt processes of social selection take place that increase the likelihood that persons who can handle or who enjoy conflict and ambiguity fill roles where these conditions are especially likely to occur. But however they are handled, the endemic nature of these stressful conditions is incontrovertible. In a U.S. national survey of 725 persons representing that part of the labor force employed during the spring of 1961, about half the respondents reported that they were caught in the middle between two conflicting persons or factions: in 88 per cent of these cases at least one of the persons involved was an organizational superior of the respondent. Almost half of all respondents reported work overload, that is, conflict among tasks or problems in setting priorities. Four forms of ambiguity were reported as particularly troublesome: uncertainty about the way one's superior evaluates one's work, about opportunities for advancement, about scope for responsibility, and about the expectations of others regarding one's performance. The difficulties people had with their organizational roles increased as conflict and ambiguity increased. On the other hand, ambiguities in such areas can be worked into defensive attitudes and ideologies that function to protect self-esteem. In the study just described, personality dimensions mediated significantly the degree to which a given intensity of objective (situational) conflict was experienced as a strain by the respondent. The effects are also mediated by the helpfulness or otherwise of colleague relations. The authors distinguished between core problems located principally in the objective environment (on which they concentrated): mismatches between the requirements of a role and the capacities of the occupant; and difficulties that are primarily intrapsychic but are acted out in the work environment. But all these intermesh, as core problems are succeeded or elaborated by derivative problems, that is, those created by the individual's attempts to cope with the core problem. Tensions arising from difficulties in work roles are not necessarily expressed wholly in those roles but may manifest themselves elsewhere in the total array of roles we all fill—as husband, father; sibling, friend, or citizen.

Intergroup conflict is a standing feature of work situations in contemporary society. Organizations are arenas of constant struggle between individuals and groups for status, power, resources, and higher shares of the collective output, in the course of which the parties seek to overcome, injure, neutralize, or eliminate their rivals. In relations between managements and workers, strikes are the most conspicuous examples of such conflicts, but they appear also in such less organized forms as work limitation, slowdowns, waste, labor turnover, absenteeism or, on the management side, overstrict discipline and discriminatory dismissals. While vertical conflicts between managements and workers arouse most public attention, this type of opposition is only one of many. What we conventionally call management is divided into a variety of subcategories and subgroups whose interests, outlook, and aspirations differ from and compete with each other. Nor are employees a homogeneous general class. They are divided into many varieties of occupation that struggle against each other for rewards, recognition, and precedence, just as many of them struggle against management. In the large, modern, complex organizations a particularly prominent form of intergroup conflict is connected with division into groups of colleagues each responsible for a share of the work: the development of occupational identities based on life investment plays a key part in the acuteness of such conflicts. Conflict is typically contained in the work organizations of advanced industrial countries, rather than bursting out in its more destructive forms, because the parties usually have other overriding interests in common and because lines of cleavance are multiple, so that it is not in the interests of the parties to press any one division to its logical end.

Conflict can confer benefits on members of organizations and on those whom they serve by facilitating change, enabling alliances to be formed, providing groups with a sense of identity, bringing problems to the attention of higher authorities, clarifying expectation, correcting imbalances in reciprocity and power, mobilizing energy, clearing the air of simmering trouble, and allowing hostile impulses to be diverted outward. From a wide, societal point of view, conflict is not a pathological phenomenon to be understood as the desperate efforts of a deprived and discontented people, but a normal aspect of "antagonistic cooperation"[1] in a competitive society in which groups cooperate but at the same time use their power to influence the outcomes of that cooperation to their greater benefit.

At the same time conflict confronts groups and individuals with breakdowns in their capacity to cooperate and to control their impulses, substitutes warfare as a motive or basis for association, blunts judgment about the behavior of oneself and others, encourages unrealistic beliefs and ideologies, reinforces self-doubt, provides a rationale for dishonesty or opportunism, and results for some in loss of power, esteem, income, or even employment. Even though structural forces and social processes provide the foundations or causes of conflicts, these tend to become personalized in the form of criticisms of the integrity, competence, and motivations of the individuals actively concerned. Since conflict is endemic in social life and inescapable in the organizational and occupational affairs of complex economic systems, it is a source of constant or intermittent stress in the work experience of most adults.

The individual's relationship with his organization appears partly to be replacing or displacing personal contacts. For many people that relationship comes to constitute one of the main sources of continuity in their life experience: while this can be argued to confer meaning and identity, there is clearly also a risk that people will become unduly dependent on their employing organizations and will play out on the organizational stage the strong emotions otherwise reserved for more private social relations.

The nature of work has changed appreciably during the past few decades. Physical tasks are increasingly being relegated to machines and physical labor is being displaced by mental effort. The occupational skills of a person may have to change often during his lifetime or may become altogether outdated. Education and training, either formal or informal, are becoming continuing processes or matters of repeated injection/ application as work processes and systems change. Employers have become active in the educational and training process. Large employers are involved in a process of secondary socialization of their members: personality and identity are not formed once and for all in childhood, and at least their external manifestations continue to be actively reshaped in adulthood, largely through the deliberate efforts of employers.

With the rapid introduction of new technologies, certain older occupations disappear and new ones emerge, for example, those of systems analyst and computer programmer. This process reduces certainty in occupational planning, introducing new occupational routes less standardized or predictable than the old and increasing the diversity of alternatives. New dangers and risks in occupational investments accompany the creation of new opportunities.

The bureaucratization of work and the rapid introduction of new occupations and techniques have contributed to changes (and possibly tensions) in the relations of younger persons to older. The career arrangements of bureaucracies place the young (even those with the latest technical skills) at the mercy of the older, putting the power to set norms and make decisions into the hands of the middle-aged.

Occupational roles have attached differences in social status, with professional workers and senior businessmen ranking at the top and unskilled manual occupations at the bottom. The higher the level of the occupation, the higher the morale of the person.

It is widely thought desirable to try to move up the occupational ladder, either during one's own lifetime (which is highly unusual) or from one's father's occupational status, and to help one's children move up from one's own occupation. Persons in a wide variety of occupational roles would prefer higher-status roles or may have aspired to higher-status roles that they have failed to achieve. Adaptation to such a situation, in the form of scaling down of ambition, can be expected in a large proportion of cases, partly because of the prevalence of this condition and the inevitable development of defensive ideologies that help to rationalize lack of achievement. But equally one can expect some less socially and personally "adjustive" reactions, such as deviant ways of gaining goals, retreat, or rebellion.

When comparisons were made of the mental health of men at different occupational levels, from white-collar workers through skilled workers, semiskilled workers, and low- level production workers, mental health was found to vary consistently with level, with more problems reported at the lower levels. It is not altogether clear, however, how far this is a direct result of factory work (and therefore possibly transient) or how far a consequence of pre-job characteristics, such as low education and downward mobility, or of such factors as low income and poor housing.

Notes

[1] This phrase derives from W. G. Sumner.

Differences in Occupational Cultures

Probably the most important dividing line between social categories in Western society today is that between blue-collar workers and white-collar workers. These labels connote profound differences not only in occupational experience but also more generally in the quality of one's personal and social life, the opportunities one is likely to be able to make available to one's children, the values to which one adheres (including those involved in bringing up children), and the model of society that one holds.

The major factors that determine which occupational category a person will enter are the social class (largely occupational class) of his parents, the number of years of formal education he has had, the size of his family, and the attitudes of the family toward education. Of these factors the strongest is one's own education, although the effects on one's progress of both education and social origin decrease in importance over time relatively to what has happened in one's career. Important handicaps to career advance are having a broken family (which affects both the husband and male offspring), having many siblings, or coming from a family not favorably disposed toward education.

Where mobility (either upward or downward) is appreciable, the mobile person experiences problems in his interpersonal relations and social identifications. Mobile persons are not liable to be closely integrated with persons either in their former or present social class in regard to life style and reciprocal influence. Mobile persons are more apt to be prejudiced against minorities and more apt to be preoccupied with their health; these attitudes may reasonably be interpreted as evidence of felt insecurity.

Intergenerational mobility is apt to create sharper discontinuities, particularly between the type of culture experienced in childhood and adulthood. Because of the increased importance of professionalism, educational selection divides children into separate educational streams with different occupational potentialities and consigns them to different social fates and life styles. When the children of professionals are not successful enough in their education to achieve the occupational level of their parents, participation in a different culture, possibly disvalued and probably more localized, is their likely social destiny.

Blue-Collar Workers

Operatives

Persons who enter blue-collar occupations have not normally had a great deal of systematic vocational guidance and are not well equipped with information to help in their occupational choices, for instance, in estimating the probable fate of various industries. They tend to enter occupations yielding relatively high short-term earnings but having relatively little opportunity for further learning or scope for advancement. This is particularly important in view of the binding character of most early occupational commitments. Many of the requisite skills are acquired in the course of the work itself and are derived from immediate work colleagues: allegiance to the work group and adherence to group norms and standards of output become a necessary condition for learning and for pleasant or tolerable social relations while at work.

A good deal of the work of persons in this sector is simple, monotonous, or boring and may consist of repetitive operations on physical objects. It may offer little scope for affirming personal competence (in a way that gives the worker feedback on his effectiveness); tasks may not be closely related to self-identity; and there may be little scope for achievement in the sense of recognition by others of the worth of one's contribution.

The context of the work may involve isolation from what is felt to be the heart of the organizational operation, a struggle to maintain or increase autonomy or control over working conditions, and effort to maintain and gain power vis-a-vis other occupational groups and particularly vis-a-vis managerial groups.

In an early industrial research classic, 180 representative workers were interviewed in their homes about their employment in one of the most modern automobile assembly lines in the world. Ninety percent of them expressed a dislike of the many jobs in the plant characterized by mechanical pacing and repetitiveness. A large number wanted jobs that lacked these characteristics. The mass production characteristic most disliked was mechanical pacing. Workers in unskilled jobs tended to devaluate themselves. The work often demanded "surface mental attention"; that is, it required a high degree of attention but was not intellectually demanding, thus being conducive to boredom. The research workers found that work arrangements denied to all but a few opportunities for a team relationship with other workers. Ability to interact was also limited by noise, speed of the line, and the amount of physical energy demanded.

The combination of the content and context of manual work is considered often to be alienating in that working conditions may foster powerlessness (the feeling that one is an object controlled and manipulated by others or by an impersonal system); self-estrangement (occupation is not experienced as constituting personal identity in an affirmative way); isolation (the feeling of being in, but not of, society, a sense of remoteness from the large social order, an absence of loyalty to intermediate collectivities); and meaninglessness (individual roles are not seen as fitting into a total system of goals of a group, organization, community, or society) .9

This is not a complete picture. There are many kinds of occupation and skill and varieties of working conditions in the blue-collar band. There is a large variety of technologies, each offering different opportunities for learning, effort, social relations, and satisfaction.

Workers of all grades have a great capacity for adapting themselves to the levels of satisfaction actually available in their jobs and for adapting even to the fact that few satisfactions (apart from income) may be available on the job and must be found elsewhere. In surveys relatively few describe themselves as acutely dissatisfied. Persons at the same occupational level vary widely in the extent to which their self-esteem is affected by the work they do; this depends on their relative investments in a wider range of human satisfactions.

Meaning can be introduced into jobs and job contexts found boring or unsatisfactory by those performing them. This is done, for example, by elaborating the movements required, by unofficial exchanges of duties between workers, by working to targets defined by the worker himself or by groups of workers, by introducing social rituals or games, or by thwarting supervisors and managerial groups. Colleagues often unwittingly collaborate with each other to use their relationships to express feelings and attitudes (both positive and negative) not strictly related to their work situation. Institutions can develop that act as defense mechanisms against tasks in a work system that arouse anxiety; an example is the depersonalization of patients, overelaborate division of labor, and ritualization of duties that occur in hospitals.

Persons in manual occupations grow up in subcultures in which expectations of satisfaction from work may not be high and the instrumental aspects of work are emphasized. Satisfaction with a particular job docs not depend purely on the quality of the work experience but on the relation between that experience, the expectations of the worker, and his assessment of the alternatives realistically open to him.

Once they have become established in their occupations the job aspirations of blue-collar workers arc typically not high, and their definitions of what constitutes success have to be judged by job needs as they perceive them, that is, largely in terms of security of employment and reasonableness of hours, colleague- ship, and supervision. On these criteria blue- collar jobs have their own typical sources of anxiety and stress. Such jobs are less secure than others; the posts held by an individual typically are not related to each other in an orderly sequence; and earnings do not rise concurrently with increasing family needs, being related more to strength, skill, and speed than to the improvements in judgment, experience, or to the capacity for looking after others that is generally accepted to come with age. The industrial worker is more subject to occupational vicissitudes than persons in more skilled or senior posts; is likely to experience or perceive randomness in occupational success; is likely to fear machines and technological improvements for their possible effects on him; is not likely to see a close connection between ability, effort, and success; and is prone to develop a philosophy of life that attributes such success to luck, pull, discrimination, or the power of others in a better position to manipulate society. A distinct ideology of the underdog or underprivileged worker expresses hopelessness, resignation, and unwillingness to believe that one matters as much as other people and that one's needs and wishes will be taken into account.

In studies of the mental health of industrial workers it is reported that a large proportion suffer from "poor life adjustment." The mental health of these workers is reported to vary significantly with situational factors, chief among which is the opportunity that work offers for the use of their abilities and for associated feelings of interest, sense of accomplishment, personal growth, and self-respect. Mental health is apparently also affected, though less appreciably, by financial stress; pace, intensity, and repetitiveness of work; the quality of supervision and personal relations on the job; opportunities for advancement and improved social status. Mental health is apt to be poorer where plants are large, a high proportion of employees are at a low level of education and skill, and personnel policies and services are below average. Mental health tends to be poorer as job level falls. Men performing routine semiskilled work experience general dissatisfaction, have a narrow range of spare-time activities, and have relatively little devotion to larger social purposes. Self-esteem is especially low in the less skilled.

In most advanced industrial countries a majority or substantial proportion of workers are affiliated to trade unions that seek to protect and advance their economic and related interests. The relationship of the individual with the union generally bulks larger as he comes to scale down his aspirations, settles for a steady job, and relies on the union to protect and advance his interests in the employment relationship and in competition with other occupational groups. In such cases the worker adjusts realistically to the fact that his mobility aspirations are more likely to be realized through his children. Ambivalence toward union membership and participation continues among those who remain ambitious to rise into the ranks of management.

The sheer size of modern industrial organizations combined with the existence of inevitably competing interests creates the occasion for the intervention of unions to deal with problems of disputes, fairness, and grievances; only in small firms it is possible to deal effectively with such matters through personal relationships. In their relations with unions, American workers appear to value most highly the job security and the protection from the dangers of wage reductions, arbitrary treatment, and deterioration of working conditions that they derive from membership.

American workers tend to have different expectations of the employer and the union. Acute conflicts in loyalty are most likely to occur in the organizing stage of unionism where ties of loyalty to the employer have to be broken for a union to be formed. In some cases the worker has little use for either employer or union, viewing both as evils to be tolerated and the whole work situation as unrewarding. But these workers appear to be greatly outnumbered in the United States by those who have no basic quarrel with the organization of industry and society and look to the union for a more equitable distribution of business income and for insurance against improper treatment.

Supervisors and Foremen

Supervisory positions have advantages over lower level jobs. Basic wage rates are higher; earnings are more regular since they do not depend on hours worked per week; status is higher in both factory and community; and promotion is known to be generally on the shop floor from among equals on the basis of demonstrated merit.

At its highest this role has been described as mediation between the rigidities and impersonalities of command and the infinite varieties of human nature, and as safeguarding of individual human dignity. It is around the supervisor that the formal instrumental pressures of managerial systems and the informal "communal" aspects of shop floor work life have to mesh.

A review of empirical studies has shown that greater job satisfaction exists among supervisory personnel than among workers. In a research project all 55 production foremen in the same plant were interviewed. On the whole and in spite of rough times, difficulties, and frustrations, the foremen liked their jobs, their employing organization, their economic rewards, and the challenges of a dynamic work environment. But real dissatisfaction existed and real problems stemmed from the technical environment and the organization of work. The conveyor belt did not substitute mechanical compulsion for human supervision. It did not solve the foreman's major problems of maintaining quality and keeping the line manned. Combined with repetitiveness it created its own problems of adjustment and morale among subordinates. To be successful with his men the foreman had to absorb pressure from many sources and still not become a symbol of pressure to his men. The foremen felt they needed help from their managements, and this was the main criterion for evaluating managerial colleagues. The foreman's main way of keeping up productivity was by keeping the line manned, but absenteeism (partly prompted by the assembly line) often frustrated this aim. The foreman was exposed to the fact that those who experience compulsions associated with "nonhuman" or "mechanical" methods are apt to accuse the agents of those compulsions of being inhuman themselves. The essence of the foreman's job was doing something different every minute.

Intermediate leaders are subject to different demands from above and below—typically demands for productivity (or its equivalent) from above and for human consideration from below—and hence are liable to actual or potential conflict in their behavior. In the U.S. Army during World War II, the noncommissioned officer was valued from above for "being a strong military leader" and from below for "being a good fellow." Ratings of foremen by superiors and subordinates have been found to be inversely correlated, with a tendency for those who are well thought of by one group to be badly thought of by the other. The supervisor must uphold the organizational standards while at the same time retaining the cooperative attitudes of subordinates. He is dependent on his subordinates both for his own reputation with his superiors and for the daily social interaction that makes work situations pleasurable or tolerable. If he does not collude with subordinates in circumventing unpopular rules, his personal position may become untenable. The supervisor may have to choose between "riding" his men or being "ridden" by his own superiors; he has to carry heavy responsibility; he has to make decisions.

In the vertical information flow of the organization, he has to keep his superiors informed about what is going on without reporting in a way that brings criticisms upon either himself or his subordinates. He is likely to be bypassed by subordinates talking to other supervisors or to union representatives about what is going on in his section. The foreman acts as the work group's intermediary with parallel work groups as well as with intermediaries. Given the demand of subordinates for consideration, one can assume ambivalence in the attention of the foreman to external tasks. He operates in a context in which he is expected to get results, but the results of his section depend on the cooperativeness of his subordinates and the largely independent activities of senior colleagues whom he does not control.

As a consequence of increased specialization, the foreman is surrounded today by a dozen (other) bosses, each a technical or staff man who has taken away a different segment of what used to be the supervisory job.

The contemporary supervisor is expected to be knowledgeable about a wide range of matters (including labor contracts and laws, company policy and regulations, technological processes, training methods) although he may well have come up the hard way and not have had much formal education. Nor may he be well prepared for the managerial side of his role: workers at the bottom of the corporate hierarchy learn to combat authority or to accept it, not how to exercise it or how to mediate between factions.

For the majority of supervisors little lies ahead in the way of promotion, since they do not possess the educational requisites for white-collar or managerial rank. Desk work may not in any case be attractive, or the entry into "polite society" may be embarrassing.

White-Collar Workers

Within the white-collar band new entrants experience some similar difficulties to blue-collar workers in occupational search and job establishment, although their vocational guidance facilities at school are almost certainly better. They have insufficient knowledge of what is involved in different occupations. They experience difficulty in estimating the prospects of different occupations, organizations, and industries. On the other hand, their preoccupations lie more with deciding what to do than with getting an acceptable job.

They may have to build a view of their capacities and occupational life chances through a series of rejections at selection procedures. They spend an amount of time choosing between options that is disproportionate to the relatively small investment of time made in generating options. Anxiety to get settled, to be an accepted member of the world of work leads to premature job crystallization, often with subsequent regret as the binding character of early commitments is realized. But compared with blue-collar workers, white-collar and executive workers in bureaucracies enter well-defined channels, and their steps thereafter are prescribed, visible, well-regulated, and supervised. Executives are helped to develop in ways not normally available to other grades of workers.

Like blue-collar workers, the white-collar and executive occupational classes value security, continuity, interaction with others, autonomy, and duties that enable them to maintain and build self-respect, test and affirm their competence, and provide scope for achievement. Like these other categories, they are resources available to their senior management and experience the pressures of working to standards imposed by others. But they are usually able to take for granted the security, continuity, and adequacy of income that are problematic for the blue-collar man. Their problems lie rather in whether they can exercise a relatively high measure of autonomy, in whether their personal resources are being well used, or whether they can identify as their own and render visible to others the contributions they make to collective efforts in which the impact of any individual is diffuse and hard to specify. Work tasks are more central to personal identity in this group, so that expectations from the work situation are high and dissatisfaction or frustration especially painful. The incorporation of work tasks into the self and a high measure of identification with the employing organization makes life satisfaction highly dependent on the work situation and career progress.

While the blue-collar worker has to tolerate the risk that he may be regarded as expendable in times of economic stringency, the white-collar worker has to tolerate a different form of insecurity and potential strain, namely, that flowing from high dependence on one employer. His skills are only partly technical but are also largely his expertise in the administrative and political processes of his own organization. A common situation is that the executive becomes heavily invested in, dependent on, and committed to one employer and is in a poor position to seek alternative employment should he experience strain or come to dislike his work situation.

Persons at higher occupational status levels report greater satisfaction with their work than those at lower levels; satisfaction seems to arise from the very fact of being in an occupation that ranks higher than others, and this has a halo effect on other aspects of the occupation and the work it involves. White- collar workers have higher expectations of their work and, in general, more sources of satisfaction. The executive and the professional have more control than junior grades over their time, the pace at which they work, and their technological and social environment, and relative freedom from hierarchical authority, at least in the way of direct surveillance. They have the opportunities to extend themselves, to define or influence their roles in accordance with their capacities and inclinations, to exercise judgment in regard to priorities among tasks. Their work contributes to their self-esteem and can be integrated into their nonwork activities. This contrasts with the operative who may see no connection between what he does as a way of earning a living and what sort of person he is.

Executives and technical specialists at a wide range of levels have their needs for security and for social interaction met, but satisfactions in esteem, autonomy, and self-actualization increase as rank rises. Among equals in managerial rank the content of duties apparently matters: line managers report more satisfaction in their jobs than staff managers, especially in regard to esteem and self-actualization."

Substantial differences exist between blue- collar and white-collar definitions of success. Emphasis on achievement in one's job and career appears particularly in nonmanual occupations, and emphasis on economic security appears particularly in manual occupations. Movement up the administrative hierarchy becomes in itself a criterion of success for the executive, a criterion whose significance is apparently maintained for a high proportion of the work life even though objective opportunities for promotion actually decline.

Clerical Workers and Lower-Level Managers

The modern office and its staff are an outgrowth of large-scale industry. When industry was conducted on a small scale, offices were correspondingly small, there were relatively few office employees, they were appreciably better educated than blue-collar workers and in close contact with management. With the subsequent growth in size of organizations, in finance invested, in government controls and taxation of industry, in procedures for collecting personal taxes through employers, and in unionism, there has been a great growth of accountability, recording, and paper work. The numbers of office workers has increased greatly.

U.S. studies have emphasized that increased costs have led to the rationalization of office work and changed roles for the office worker. The roles of bookkeeper, clerk, and secretary have been fragmented, become more routinized and to some extent more mechanized—in this way following somewhat the same course as shop floor roles. Nevertheless, important differences exist in the connection of the duties of the office worker with abstract symbols rather than physical materials, in the clerk's physical proximity and access to members of the managerial hierarchy, in cleaner and quieter physical working conditions, and in the opportunity to wear clothing also appropriate outside the workplace.

In regard to work satisfaction, one of the few exceptions to the rule that reported satisfaction decreases as level in the occupational pyramid lowers is that skilled manual workers are slightly more satisfied than rank-and-file white-collar workers. This is found in the United States, Germany, and the U.S.S.R.

Over the past few decades the salaries of U.S. office workers and bluecollar workers have converged, partly through rationalization of work, partly through wider educational opportunities, partly through the greater strength of blue-collar unions. Office workers seem to have been put in a position of status ambiguity, a difference arising between their status claims and aspirations, on the one hand, and their objective position and the reluctance of blue-collar workers to concede their superiority, on the other.

Strains among office workers and the lowest levels of management are thought to arise from salaries that are too low to finance the middle-class aspirations characteristic of these employees and from relative status decline. To the extent that office work becomes mechanized one can expect increasing strains similar to that experienced by the operative confronted with technological advances.

In Britain the basic skill of literacy used to set the clerk apart from the working man and give him a foothold on the lowest rung of the middle-class ladder. Although he lacked the income and security of the middle-class person, this is where his identification lay. Status considerations were powerful. But the connection with middle-class status has been altered by social and economic changes. Economic power has shifted toward organized labor and educated people have become less scarce. There has been a fall in the desirability and prestige of clerical work in the eyes of other occupational groups.

The clerk belongs neither to the middle class nor the working class. In social background, education, working conditions, proximity to authority, and opportunity for upward mobility, clerks in Britain can still perhaps claim a higher status than most manual workers. But using other criteria such as income and skill, they may be rated lower, or no different, by manual workers. Clerical workers are also divided among themselves or uncertain on the question of where they stand in the social hierarchy.

The position of clerical workers and lower- level managers has recently been particularly affected by the introduction of electronic data processing. Persons in these grades have tended to be especially security-minded, and many have worked under conditions more stable than those of either bluecollar workers or executives. The disorganization and reorganization associated with change to EDP may have found them less ready in personality and experience to meet the demands for adjustment. The nature of clerical jobs is changing with the automation of office processes. The most routine jobs are being eliminated and work pace is becoming more closely tied to machines, so that absence and lateness matter more. While the office worker still has more freedom than the blue-collar worker to leave his workplace or to vary his production level, more specific work quotas have been imposed. Opportunities for promotion may have been somewhat reduced, and some shift work has been introduced. There is lower tolerance for errors, which become transmitted far through the system and are more visible to superiors and customers. With the rationalization of the work system, each job gains significance in the continuity of the overall process and the individual becomes more accountable for his actions. With automation a proportion of jobs may be eliminated or changed radically. While new jobs are created, the persons displaced may not be able to fill them or may not be easily amenable to retraining.

In a British study drawing on data from nine firms that had introduced computers, it was found that this and concomitant reorganization were experienced as a threat to staff security. There was much initial anxiety, even where little redundancy ensued. Staff often had to be redeployed. It proved difficult to avoid reducing the status and salary of staff in the 45 to 55 age group, particularly if they had held supervisory positions. In the clerical area there was a greater concentration of responsibility and a need for more staff of high intelligence: those associated with running computers had to be able to master complicated new skills. In some firms junior managerial roles also changed, sometimes only eliminating routine, but in other cases involving transfers from reduced departments and loss of status. Not all the results of the new computer installations were negative. Many of the younger clerical workers were attracted toward machine work, which seemed to promise greater interest and more promotion opportunities than the "elementary" clerical duties they were performing.

Middle-Level Managers

A review of empirical studies has shown that median satisfaction with jobs is higher for managerial than nonmanagerial personnel and that satisfaction increases with echelon level within management.

The middle manager's work is carried out in a highly "political" context; he is part of a constant struggle for relative power, autonomy, and influence over the way the overall enterprise is run, not only between individuals, but also between departments and occupational groups. The acuteness of these struggles derives largely from the investments made by the persons involved in their occupational training and experience and from the difficulty of radical occupational shifts in adulthood— particularly among those wishing to protect their status as higher-level managers or technical specialists.

The middle-level manager's situation is deeply affected by expectations (both his own and others) that he should climb up the administrative hierarchy. He has two tasks to perform simultaneously: that of carrying out organizational tasks in cooperation with colleagues and that of facilitating his upward rise. Most organizational tasks are carried out by groups that develop solidarity, shared definitions of their mission and status, and shared conceptions of how they should relate to other task groups, subordinates, and superiors. Therefore, the individual must be an acceptable colleague on easy terms with equals, prepared to give credit to their contributions and to refrain from pressing his own claims to special consideration and merit. But if he is to advance it is also necessary that he differentiate himself from his peers and convey his potential ability to distance himself enough to view their organizational contribution objectively or, if required, to control it from a position of greater authority. Both task performance and career building make high demands on interpersonal competence. Discussion of this topic usually emphasizes the need for the executive to conform, to represent himself as similar to others. But the task is more correctly viewed as a wider form of self-management, involving both a measure of conformity and a capacity for discreet and acceptable differentiation.

The character of a great deal of executive work is diffuse and is not subject to clear-cut criteria of adequacy. This makes assessment of the executive's competence dependent on evaluation by colleagues, of which evaluation by seniors is the most crucial. Because of the absence of objective evidence of performance and the difficulty, where there is an ascertainable output, of establishing that it is a direct consequence of a particular executive's input, evaluation of the executive tends to acquire a personal quality, so that he gets evaluated on such grounds as enthusiasm, confidence, assertiveness, patience, and cooperativeness alongside technical competence, knowledge, and capacity for problem solving. The personal component of this evaluation is accentuated by the fact that appraisal by superiors covers not only his performance but also his potential: an aspect that necessarily brings into issue the amount of flexibility and capacity for growth and change in his personality relative to the more senior roles in the organization. It is common practice for large organizations to inform their executives in appraisal interviews of their personal strengths and weaknesses in relation to their careers; the rationale is that this will increase the likelihood that the person will alter in a direction likely to bring greater organizational rewards, with resultant benefits to both the employer and himself. The extent of defensiveness in appraisees and the protective distortions that occur imply that the interviews are stressful events at least for the appraisee and possibly tor the appraiser also. The executive faces a unique life situation in that he cannot escape or by-pass an organizational mirror that confronts him with the image held of him by his most important seniors.

He is commonly subject to personal dependence on one or more sponsors, persons with whom he has an interdependent relationship of reciprocal support. The executive's career becomes linked with that of his sponsor or sponsors, increasing his chances of rising as his sponsor gains status and influence, but simultaneously increasing his vulnerability as his sponsor's career goes through its own vicissitudes.

A systematic connection between rank, conflict, and tension has been found in a national survey, with the maximum of conflict occurring at the upper-middle levels of management. The research workers interpret this as partly a consequence of the still unfulfilled mobility aspirations of middle management, in contrast with the better actualized aspirations of top management. The greatest pressure is evidently directed to a person from others who are in the same department as himself, who are his superiors in a hierarchy and who are sufficiently dependent on his performance to care about his adequacy without being so completely dependent as to be inhibited in making their demands known.

The tapering of the administrative hierarchy and the definition of success as movement combine to produce career disappointment in many executives. Some adapt fairly comfortably to their work situation or are helped to do so by the personnel institutions of their organizations. The disappointed person may be able to call on his individual defense mechanisms in the sense that he can tell himself that he has not been given a fair chance or that he would not stoop to the methods used by others to secure advancement. He is commonly helped by the existence of shared group ideologies, developed with colleagues in the same position as himself, whose central theme is that personal merit is not the main determinant of success. Some are able to find compensations in other aspects of their lives. External compensatory roles may include devotion (or more devotion) to familial, recreational, political, or social service pursuits. Role segmentation may usefully insulate compartments of one's life against failure and disappointment in others. One form of (negative) response is to turn "sour" in relations with the employing organization by withdrawing enthusiasm, good will, and vitality from one's work role, complying with the formal requirements of the role but withdrawing identification from it.

A key factor in career disappointment is that persons come to base their self-identity on the assumption that they will in due course come to occupy certain organizational roles more senior than their own. A career disappointment can then come to constitute a disturbance in self-conception, involving the necessity to reassess or reclassify oneself, and an embarrassing withdrawal of the image of the prospective self that one may have held out to intimates. Seniors may be felt to have betrayed one. Personal and familial sacrifices may have been made in the vain pursuit of illusory occupational goals. Internal readjustment may be painful, and in seeking to justify to those closest to him his revised expectations and evaluations, the person may have to perform a stressful about-face and express himself in transparent rationalizations.

Technical Specialists

Line managers report themselves to be more satisfied in their jobs than staff managers, mainly because the latter feel they have to be directed by others.

Technical specialists complain that they are subjected to administrative routines and controls that are alien to their notions of reciprocal control by equals; that they are overconstrained by considerations of practicality and profitability and have too little opportunity for work of long-term importance; that undue secrecy is placed on their work, on relations with colleagues in other organizations, and on publication; that they are appraised and managed by nonspecialists who do not understand their work; and that their rewards and promotion chances are inferior to those of line administrators. A distinction has been drawn between cosmopolitans and locals: this differentiates persons whose major commitment is toward their discipline and to colleagues wherever they are located from those whose more abiding interests and personal loyalty reside with their employing organization. While important conflicts no doubt exist, most people are unlikely to lie at one extreme or another.

Accommodative mechanisms arise or are developed to reduce strain, to forestall and to settle actual or incipient conflict. In general, bureaucratic organizations are adapting themselves to the high proportion of technical specialists they now employ. Special roles are created for specialists in segregated departments, for example, research and development. Special administrative arrangements can be made to allow for colleague control in project teams whose leadership shifts in accordance with the dominant specialty involved. Specialist leaders are appointed who have qualifications and interests in both the disciplines involved and in "organizational" needs, and who can mediate between the technical specialists and superiors. Leave can be arranged to provide sufficient contact with outside colleagues. Dual career ladders have sometimes been created so that specialists can improve their prestige, income, and facilities without giving up their specialties. Those people who are most insistent on pure science and academic freedom are apt to avoid careers in the applied research departments of large organizations. Even in the most enthusiastic and tenacious research, worker compromise and adaptation will occur.

Industrial research provides appropriate positions for those technical specialists (who may be a substantial proportion) who are distinctly interested in their subject and feel it is an important part of their lives, but who are unwilling to have it as the dominating factor in their lives.

Some studies have concentrated on the organizational scientists who remain anxious to retain their full status as members of the scientific profession. They have to span two areas, since consolidation of their organizational positions is a prerequisite for gaining and maintaining recognition by external colleagues. Only a positive evaluation of their own work by their organizational superiors will give them the facilities and resources they need for successful research. At the same time they become dependent on having assistants and subordinates who become counters in their own career success.

Senior Administrators

Taking various dimensions of job satisfaction separately, a review of U.S. research shows that within management security and social affiliation needs are equally met, but that the needs for esteem, autonomy, and selfactualization are better met at each higher level. The phenomenon of greater job satisfaction at higher levels of management is not confined to the United States; in a cross-cultural investigation of managerial attitudes in 14 countries, higher levels of management on the whole reported that their needs were better satisfied in their jobs.

Seniors are more exposed and vulnerable to criticism than middle-level executives or blue-collar workers. The less senior members of an organization are better protected by the narrower specification of their responsibilities and are in a better position to discharge their obligations by adhering to the instructions issued to them. Their errors are usually less visible and their rights more likely to be defended by formal collective associations or their informal equivalent.

Senior administrators may experience frustrations from the limits to their behavior set by the crystallization of organizational practices over time by laws, regulations, and agreements covering the roles involved in the organization, the means by which these must be filled or vacated, and the conditions under which personnel may be employed or dismissed.

While it is one of the tasks of the senior administrative group to initiate changes, such changes are liable to alter the existing distribution of power and prestige. A tension can be set up between following out the logic of an organizational change and accepting the implications that the change will have for one's own position and behavior.

In the earlier phases of his career the senior administrator will probably first have developed and practiced some form of specialist expertise, then have combined this with responsibility for a group of subordinates. At the most senior levels opportunities for direct development and practice of such special knowledge decrease, and usually the transition has to be made to being a generalist. The security of acknowledged specialist knowledge and techniques is given up for the exercise of judgment and wisdom on issues on which there is no clear-cut right and wrong and where one is more exposed to challenge.

The senior administrator has to steer a path between the advice of a variety of rival specialist colleagues. He has to show that he respects the views of each but may, nevertheless, have to act in ways that advance the interests of some and obstruct those of others. In order to maintain objectivity in his judgments he will find it necessary to maintain distance from previously close colleagues, with probable feelings of isolation or loneliness. His wife may also find herself in a similar position in relation to the families of her husband's colleagues. The administrator carries responsibility for large sums of money, large numbers of people, and farreaching decisions but does so in a chronic state of uncertainty, since knowledge of the relevant facts, including future events, is always imperfect.

The roles that senior administrators play at the top of an organization have more scope for variation and for idiosyncratic interpretation than those lower down. This is largely because it is the function of the senior executive person or executive group to define organizational priorities. If, as is usual in large organizations, a number of people are involved, either formally or informally, some accommodation must take place between them in regard to relative power and duties. How things turn out will clearly depend on a combination of formal position, personality, traditions of colleagueship and popular support among subordinates and, perhaps, sponsors and shareholders. Interpersonal relations with close colleagues will bulk very large in the psychological life space. There will be a further division of labor in the psychological sense that each senior administrator will tend to perform particular psychological functions or have these projected on to him by subordinates. One might, for instance, symbolize instrumental purposes, another the supportive "maintenance" activities that also appear necessary in organizational functioning. A study of a hospital has identified the allocation of these roles among a colleague group of three and implied that, apart from objective task definition, problems may arise if administrators fit poorly into the psychological functions allocated to them by group processes, if they are too similar in personality, or if their own prior socialization has prepared them inadequately for these highly demanding social psychological roles.

Bibliography

Avery, R. W., "Enculturation in Industrial Research" excerpted in Glaser, B. G. (Ed.), *Organizational Careers,* Aldine, Chicago, 1968.

Barber, B., "The Sociology of the Professions," *Daedalus,* Fall 1963.

Bedrosian, H., "Managerial Obsolescence in Banking," in Lazarus, H., and Warren, K. (Eds.), *The Progress of Management,* Prentice-Hall, Englewood Cliffs, N.J., 1968.

Belbin, E., and Belbin, R. M., "New Careers in Middle Age," in Neugarten, B. L., *Middle Age and Aging,* University of Chicago Press, Chicago, 1968.

Bell, D., *Work and Its Discontents,* Beacon, Boston, 1956.

Blackburn, R. M., *Union Character and Social Class,* Batsford, London, 1967. Blau, P. M.,

"Social Mobility and Interpersonal Relations," *Am. Sociol. Rev., 21,* 1956. ___, and Duncan,

O. D., *The American Occupational Structure,* John Wiley, New York, 1967.
Blauner, R., *Alienation and Freedom: The Factory Worker and His Industry,* University of Chicago Press, Chicago, 1964.

___, "Work Satisfaction and Industrial Trends in Modern Society," in Galenson, W., and Lipset, S. M. (Eds.), *Labor and Trade Unionism: An Inter-disciplinary Reader,* John Wiley, New York, 1960.

Borow, H. (Ed.), *Man in a World of Work,* Houghton Mifflin, Boston, 1964.

Cain, L. D., "Life Course and Social Structure," in Faris, R. E. L. (Ed.), *Handbook of Modem Sociology,* Rand McNally, Chicago, 1964.
Centers, R., "Attitude and Belief in Relation to Occupational Stratification," *J. Soc. Psychol.,* 27.159 185,1948.

Chinoy, E., *The Automobile Worker and the American Dream,* Doubleday, New York,

1955Coser, L., *The Functions of Social Conflict,* Free Press, Glencoe, 1956.

Crozier, M., *The Bureaucratic Phenomenon: An Examination of Bureaucracy in Modern*
        Organizations and Its Cultural Setting in France, University of Chicago Press, Chicago,
1964.

Dill, W. R., Hilton, T. L., and Reitman, W. R., *The New Managers: Patterns of Behaviour and*
        Development, Prentice-Hall, Englewood Cliffs, N.J., 1962.

Down, E., and Adelson, J., "Social Mobility in Adolescent Boys," *J. Abnorm. & Soc. Psychol, 56,* 1958.

Fleishman, E. A., Harris, E. F., and Burt, E., *Leadership and Supervision in Industry: An Evaluation*
of
        a Supervisory Training Programme, Ohio State University Press, Columbus, 1955.

Glaser, B. G. (Ed.), *Organizational Careers: A Source Book for Theory,* Aldine, Chicago, 1968.

____, *Organizational Scientists: Their Professional Careers,* Bobbs-Merrill, Indianapolis,

1964. ____, and Strauss, A., *Status Passage: A Formal Theory,* Aldine-Atherton, Chicago,

Goffman, E., "On Cooling the Mark Out: Some Aspects of Adaptation to Failure," *Psychiatry, 15,*
1971.   1952.

Goldthorpe, J. H., Lockwood, D., Bechhofer, F., and Platt, J., *The Affluent Worker: Industrial*
        Attitudes and Behaviour, Cambridge University Press, Cambridge, 1968.

Gouldner, A. W., "Cosmopolitans and Locals: Toward an Analysis of Latent Social Roles," *Admin.*
        Sci. Quart., 2, 1957.

____, *Patterns of Industrial Bureaucracy,* Free Press, Glencoe, 1954.

____, "The Unemployed Self," in Fraser, R. (Ed.), *Work,* Vol. 2, Penguin Books, London,

1969. Gross, E., *Industry and Social Life,* Brown, Dubuque, Iowa, 1956.

_____, *Work and Society,* Thomas Y. Crowell, New York, 1958.

Herzberg, F., Mausner, B., and Snyderman, B. B., *The Motivation to Work,* John Wiley, New York, 1959.

Hodgson, R. C., Levinson, D. J., and Zaleznik, A., *The Executive Role Constellation,* Harvard Graduate
      School of Business Administration, Cambridge, 1965.

Ingham, G. J., *Size of Industrial Organisation and Worker Behaviour,* Cambridge University Press, Cambridge, 1970.

Inkeles, A., "Industrial Man: The Relation of Status to Experience, Perception and Values," *Am. J. Sociol.,* 66:1-31, 1960.

Jennings, E. E., *Routes to the Executive Suite,* McGraw-Hill, New York, 1971.

Kahn, R. L., Wolfe, D. M., Quinn, R. P., and Snoek, J. D., *Organizational Stress: Studies in Role Conflict*
      and Ambiguity, John Wiley, New York, 1964.

Knupper, G., "Portrait of the Underdog," *Public Opinion Quart., 11,*

1947. Kohn, M. L., "Bureaucratic Man," *New Society,* October 28, 1971.
_____, "Bureaucratic Man: A Portrait and an Interpretation," *Am. Sociol. Rev.,* 36, 1971.

Kornhauser, A., *Mental Health of the Industrial Worker, A Detroit Study,* John Wiley, New York, 1965.

Kornhauser, W., *Scientists in Industry,* University of California Press, Berkeley, 1962.

Levinson, H., "Reciprocation: The Relationship between Man and Organisation," *Admin. Sci. Quart.,* 9:370-390, 1964.

Lipset, S. M., and Bendix, R., *Social Mobility in Industrial Society,* University of California Press, Berkeley, 1959.

Lockwood, D., *The Blackcoated Worker,* Unwin, London, 1958.

MacWhinney, W. R. H., and Adelman, S. R., "Mental Health of the Industrial Worker: An Analysis and Review," *Human Organization,* 25, 1966.

Mann, F. C., and Williams, L. K., "Organizational Impact of White Collar Automation," *Proceedings of Eleventh Animal Meeting, Industrial Relations Research Association,* 1958.

Marcson, S., *The Scientist in American Industry,* Harper, New York, 1960.

Menzies, I. E. P., "A Case Study in the Functioning of Social Systems as a Defence against Anxiety: A Report of a Study of the Nursing Services of a General Hospital," *Human Rel, 13,* 1960.

Merton, R. K., *Social Theory and Social Structure,* Free Press, Glencoe,

1957. Mills, C. W., *White Collar,* Oxford University Press, London, 1951.
Moore, W. E., and Tumin, M. M., "Some Social Functions of Ignorance," *Am. Sociol. Rev., 14,* 1949.

Morse, N. C., and Weiss, R. S., "The Function and Meaning of Work and the Job," *Am. Sociol. Rev.,* 20,1955.

Mumford, E., *Living with a Computer,* Institute of Personnel Management, London, 1964.

Neff, W. S., *Work and Human Behaviour,* Atherton Press, New York, 1968. Neugarten, B. L.

(Ed.), *Middle Age and Ageing,* University of Chicago Press, Chicago, 1968. Palmer, G. L.,

"Attitudes toward Work in an Industrial Community," *Am. J. Sociol., 63,* 1957.
Pellegrin, R. J., and Coates, C. H., "Executives and Supervisors. Contrasting Definitions of Career Success," *Admin. Sci. Quart., 1,* 1956-1957.

Porter, L. W., "Job Attitudes in Management," *J. Appl. Psychol., 46,* 1962; *47,* 1963; *47,* 1963.

_____, and Lawler, E. E., "Properties of Organization Structure in Relation to Job Attitudes and Job Behaviour," *Psychol. Bull., 64,* 1965.

Roethlisberger, F. J., *Man in Organization,* Harvard University Press, Cambridge, 1968.

Roy, D. F., "'Banana Time': Job Satisfaction and Informal Interaction," *Human Organization, 18,* 1959-1960.

_____, "Work Satisfaction and Social Rewards in Quota Achievement: An Analysis of Piecework," *Am. Sociol. Rev., 18,* 1953.

Schneider, E. V., *Industrial Sociology,* McGraw-Hill, New York, 1957.

Sofer, C., "Buying and Selling: A Study in the Sociology of Distribution," *Sociol. Rev., 13,*

1965. _____, *Men in Mid-Career,* Cambridge University Press, Cambridge, 1970. _____, *The*

Organisation from Within, Tavistock Publications, London, 1961.
Stouffer, S. A., Lumsdaine, A. A., Lumsdaine, M. H., Williams, R. M., Brewster Smith, M., Janis, I. L., Star, S. A., and Cottrell, L. S., *The American Soldier,* Vol. 2, *Combat and Its Aftermath,* Princeton University Press, Princeton, 1949

_____, Suchman, E. A., De Vinney, L. C., Star, S. A., and Williams, R. M., *The American Soldier,* Vol. 1, *Adjustment during Army Life,* Princeton University Press, Princeton, 1949.

Turner, A. N., and Lawrence, P. R., *Industrial Jobs and the Worker,* Harvard Graduate School of Business Administration, Cambridge, 1965.

von Mises, L., *Bureaucracy,* Yale University Press, New Haven,

1946. Vroom, V. H., *Work and Motivation,* John Wiley, New York,
Walker, C. R., and Guest, R. H., *The Man on the Assembly Line,* Harvard University
1964.   Cambridge, 1952.

___, ___, and Turner, A. N., *The Foreman on the Assembly Line,* Harvard University Press,
Cambridge, 1956.

Watson, W., "Social Mobility and Social Class in Industrial Communities," in Gluekman, M. (Ed.),
Closed Systems and Open Minds, Oliver & Boyd, London, 1964.

Wilensky, H. L., "Work, Careers and Social Integration," *Internat. Soc. Sci. J., 12,* 1960.

___, and Edwards, H., "The Skidder: Ideological Adjustments of Downward Mobile Workers,"
Am.
     Sociol. Rev., 24, 1959.

Weiss, R. S., and Riesman, D., "Social Problems and Disorganization in the World of Work," in
Merton, R. K., and Nisbet, R. A. (Eds.), *Contemporary Social Problems,* Harcourt Brace,
New York, 1961.

Zytowski, D. G., *Vocational Behaviour: Readings in Theory and Research,* Holt, Rinehart, New York,
1968.